Coconut Oil

Breakthrough

Burn the Fat, Boost Your Brain,
Build Your Hair

BJ Richards

ISBN: 978-1533468574

Disclaimer

Legal Notice: Richards Media Services, LLC and BJ Richards and the accompanying materials have used their best intention of providing correct and reliable information. The information provided is offered solely for informational purposes and is universal as so. This information is presented without contract or any type of guarantee assurance.

Richards Media Services, LLC and BJ Richards make no representation or warranties with respect to the accuracy, applicability, fitness or completeness of the contents of this book. The information contained in this book is strictly for educational purposes. Therefore, if you wish to apply ideas contained in this book, you are taking full responsibility for your actions.

Richards Media Services, LLC and BJ Richards disclaim any warranties (express or implied), merchantability, or fitness for any particular purpose. Richards Media Services, LLC and BJ Richards shall

Dedication

This book would not have been possible if not for the encouragement of the fur children who kept me laughing and helped me take a break when it was needed. Thank you Simon, Chloe, Rudy and Elsa. You kept me smelling the roses.

And to my loving daughter who is so proud of me for becoming an author.

Free Coconut Oil Recipes

You can get the follow free recipes here: http://bjrichardsauthor.com/recipe-sign-up/

They're fun to make, healthy and delicious!

- Weight-Loss-Wonder Coconut Smoothie

- Super-Satisfying Coconut Almond Smoothie

- Homemade Cinnamon-Coconut-Granola Crunch

- Tempting Fried Coconut Shrimp

- Happy-Healthy Coconut Omelet with Veggies

ALSO: Find out about my new books when they come out. Sign up at the link below:

http://bjrichardsauthor.com/newsletter-sign-up/

Contents

Introduction

You're here because you still haven't found the answers you're looking for. Maybe you want to lose those stubborn pounds, revive your brain or save your hair before it's too late.

What if there was something you could use in your regular eating that helped to:

Burn off fat, pounds and inches

Give your brain what it needs to rebuild

Repair damaged broken hair

Increase your energy

Beautify your skin

And help resolve major health issues.

Coconut oil does all that and more without you spending hundreds of dollars a month or burning up precious time running from specialist to specialist.

I've been a natural health advocate and researcher for over 30 years. Instead of you having to spend days and hours clicking on hundreds of websites and verifying countless articles, I've done the heavy lifting for you in this book. I've compiled the best most accurate information I could find and put it all into one convenient source, simplifying the jargon, sorting through the dubious and distilling out the duplicate information. Now I'm going to share that with you.

I'll teach you how to use coconut oil to lose weight and burn fat, along with secrets to help you live life with greater health, vigor and enjoyment. You'll learn what kind of coconut oil to use and why using the wrong kind of coconut oil can be disastrous for your health. Plus, you'll get health tips and beauty secrets that are simple and easy to implement, all without breaking the bank.

This book is more than just a guide about how to use coconut oil. It separates out the fact from the fiction. There are a lot of new scientific studies that have proven how effective coconut oil can be for changing and improving your health, brain function and overall resistance to illness; plus, it is now recognized as an essential weight loss aid. Don't just do something because you heard it works. Find out why so you can use coconut oil effectively for a better life.

After reading this book, you'll understand how beneficial coconut oil is for leading a healthy and energetic life and how to make that happen for yourself. People who have made coconut oil a regular part of their lives, often live many years longer than others. Not only does it have amazing effects on the health of your body organs, you can use the benefits of the coconut to help resolve skin and hair issues as well. And last but not least, its use enhances the powers of your brain.

You're going to learn about the amazing gifts of coconut oil, as well as the benefits of coconut milk and coconut water and how to use them to improve your hair, skin and overall health. You'll also discover how and why coconut milk and coconut water contribute to weight loss and boost your energy levels. I'll also include a recipe for how to make your own coconut milk for just pennies.

Dr. Oz is so impressed with coconut oil he did a 2-part series on his show entitled, "Coconut Oil Superpowers". And he's not the only medical professional and scientist to endorse coconut oil. Dr. Weil and Dr. Mercola are also proponents of the coconut and its byproducts. If these medical professionals are willing to stake their reputation on its medical and therapeutic values, then maybe it's time for all of us to take a closer look at how we can benefit personally in our daily lives.

I promise if you implement even some of these secrets and tips, you'll find yourself heading down a path of improved health and wellbeing, something you may have been seeking for years.

But you need to take action. Sitting on the sidelines hasn't helped you burn off those extra pounds or improved your brain or stopped your hair from thinning. And that's not going to change until you act. These strategies have been proven to produce long-lasting results for those that actually use them. Now is the time to improve your health, beautify your body and open yourself up to a higher level of health and happiness.

"If you do nothing, nothing is likely to happen. So DO SOMETHING!" Raymon Grace

Don't waste another day wondering what to do about great hair, rebuilding your brain and losing weight. Take control of your life now. A new healthier body awaits you. Time to enjoy the life you've created.

Brief History of Coconut Oil

How did the use of coconut oil come about? When and how have they been using it before now? Let's find out.

Coconut has gone by many names throughout the centuries. In some cultures, it was known as the 'Tree of Heaven', 'Tree of Life', or 'Nature's Super Market'. This was due to its widely known and accepted nutritional and healing qualities in the countries where it was grown and traded.

The coconut tree itself is scientifically known by 'cocos nucifera'. It was the Spanish and Portuguese that came up with the word 'coconut' back in the 16th century. The word 'coco' means "a grin" or "a monkey face". Something we commonly see every time we pick up a coconut; that cute little face smiling back at us on the outside shell.

Coconut trees do not fare well in cooler temperatures, which is why you see them growing in warm tropical climates where the soil is sandy and there is plenty of sun and rain. More than 90 countries are now known to grow and utilize coconut in their indigenous cultures. Those countries are producing close to 10.9 million tons of coconut every year.

The most valuable component of the coconut was and continues to be its oil. Not only does the coconut provide invaluable nutritional and therapeutic assets for millions, the coconut farms are providing a living for thousands and contributing to the economic structure of those 90 countries.

Coconut use has been recorded and reported for over 3900 years. I'm sure it was a wonderful asset to cultures before that, but records have not yet been found or they weren't written down. According to the records we do have there was widespread use of coconut oil, coconut meat and coconut water for nutritional and therapeutic uses, much as we use it today.

The coconut was also used in trade with countries where it does not grow and became a valuable economic asset as well. Coconut use was particularly prevalent in tropical populations such as the Polynesian Islands, most of Asia, South and Central Americas, Africa and the Indian subcontinent.

Ayurvedic medicine has recorded the use of coconut in its therapeutic traditions since 1500 BC and considers coconut to influence not only the body, but the soul and psyche as well. Even the early European explorers such as Captain Cook wrote about the popular influence of coconut oil on the Pacific cultures and the important part it played in the everyday lives of those peoples.

Coconut water became an invaluable asset during WWII. Saline was difficult to get in the medical units of the battle fields. As a substitute young green coconut water was utilized effectively for saline trickle, saving hundreds of lives. Then when the war was over, coconut oil was sold as margarine in England and as "coconut spread" in the United States.

In spite of all the many uses of coconut oil and its proven nutritional value for centuries, its popularity changed in 1954. Studies on fats came out and erroneously identified the fats in coconut oil as non-beneficial. Coconut oil was demonized because the studies did not differentiate between the different types of fats and their roles in the body.

We know now that some of the saturated fats are not only healthy, but essential for humans. At that time, they treated all types of fats the same and labeled them all as bad and unhealthy, doing a great disservice to peoples everywhere that believed and followed those erroneous findings.

Now that we understand why the old studies were wrong, let's find out the truth about why coconut oil is so good for you. How do some fats make me thin and others make me gain weight? Good questions that deserve answers next.

What About the Fat in Coconut Oil?

In this chapter we'll find out about the different kinds of fats and how they can affect you, in either a good way or a detrimental way. different treatments such as balancing hormones, blood sugar and improving energy levels.

Coconut oil is an edible fatty oil. It comes from ripe coconut meat. The oil is used throughout a number of industries including cosmetic, medical and industrial. Alternative medicine also uses coconut oil in a number of different treatments such as balancing hormones, blood sugar and improving energy levels.

While food companies have poured billions of dollars into advertising trying to make it look like hydrogenated oils are healthy for consumption, it simply is not the case. In reality these oils raise the levels of low-density lipoprotein (LDL) in the body. This is a technical term for the bad cholesterol that concerns medical professionals everywhere. Virgin coconut oil does just the opposite. It raises the levels of good cholesterol in the body, something that has been proven repeatedly.

Due to current and more advanced studies we now know that all saturated fats are not the same and coconut oil is a huge exception. Why is this? Because it contains an exceedingly large percentage of medium-chain fatty acids which are closest to those naturally found in the breast milk of humans. This is why you see coconut oil broadly used as a part of baby formulas as well as other nutritional beverages and energy bars.

Many people get turned off when they hear the word "fat". But there are good fats as well as bad fats. Coconut oil is full of medium-chain triglycerides and these fats are good for you.

The body naturally digests and uses medium-chain fatty acids more effectively than fats found in other oils. This is because they are handled in the liver, which immediately converts them to energy. That makes less strain on the pancreas, liver and entire digestive system and provides a very useable source of fuel for the body. And it enhances the retention of different nutritional supplements.

Ninety percent of coconut oil is made up from these good fats. These are not ordinary fats; they won't clog your arteries. The body needs these good fats to function properly. Medium-chain tricglycerides (MCTS) function very differently from the long-chain fatty acids found in hydrogenated oils. Fats found in hydrogenated oils are not absorbed quickly and usually get stored as fat in the body, the really stubborn kind that can take forever to get rid of.

The previous researchers didn't discover this because they were using hydrogenated coconut oil in the studies, not virgin coconut oil. Hydrogenated oils go through a process that converts all fats into unhealthy trans unsaturated fats. This is also the problem with many of the oils on the market today that are labeled as healthy. They, too, are processed hydrogenated oils that lead to a number of maladies. These hydrogenated oils create free radicals when they become heated and are known today for causing numerous health problems.

Coconut oil on the other hand, does not produce free radicals when heated. It will remain stable even at high temperatures. This is why virgin coconut oil is considered a safe oil to cook with and is utilized by many educated and health-conscious people throughout the world.

Some will argue about the proof that the saturated fat in coconut oil is beneficial. There are always two sides to every coin. However, more and more studies are showing proven results. There are, however, several studies that do prove how unbeneficial the fats in hydrogenated oils are, to the point of being labeled as detrimental to human health.

Now you know the difference between the healthy saturated fat in coconut oil and what happens in the body when you eat unhealthy hydrogenated fat. You also learned why you gain energy when you eat virgin coconut oil. But there is more than one kind of coconut oil out there. The next chapter will tell you which one you need and why.

The Only Kind of Coconut Oil to Use

This chapter is going to teach you what kind of coconut oil to look for and what kind to avoid. You'll also learn how indigenous cultures have been making their own coconut oil for centuries.

There are two broad categories of coconut oil:

1) Industrially mass produced and highly refined.

2) Fresh coconut that is much less refined. This is what we want.

By nature, coconut oil is already a refined product because the oil is inside the coconut and doesn't grow on the tree, the coconuts do. To get to the oil you have to extract it from the coconut where it is truly natural and unrefined. Which means the only true "unrefined" coconut oil is still inside the meat of the coconut and just off the tree.

The term "virgin coconut oil" came about in the early 2000s to indicate the least refined coconut oils for sale on the market. In the case of coconuts, this means not using "copra" as the starting point for extracting the coconut oil.

So what is "copra"? Copra is an industry-defined term companies in the Philippines used to refer to the dried coconut meat that has been removed from the shell and is inedible due to their processes. It has to go through further processing to produce coconut oil at this point.

In countries that produce and process coconut products, refined coconut oils are referred to as "RBD", which stands for: refined, bleached, deodorized. Bleaching is a process that removes impurities and is generally not a chemical process. Normally bleaching clay is used for the filtering. The deodorizing is done by steam so the end result is an oil with little to no odor and a bland taste.

Copra is created through a variety of methods which can be drying by sun, smoke or kiln or a combination of these drying methods. At this point the product is dirty and smoky and cannot be internally consumed. Copra is its own commodity and is often sold to coconut oil manufacturing plants, even in the United States where they refine it even further. So you can understand why you wouldn't want any coconut oil that is not "virgin coconut oil".

Food grade coconut oil means it has passed a kind of quality control test and was manufactured in a plant that is not full of contaminants and other things you don't want in or on your body.

These are the types of refined coconut oils you can find for sale:

Coconut Oil: If you don't see any type of description on the label, most likely it is RBD coconut oil. Copra-producing companies export to the United States among other countries where it is refined into a number of inedible products such as cleaning products and detergents. Since coconut oil has become so popular, some of these companies are now starting to produce and sell coconut oil for internal consumption. These cheaper products are most likely mass produced with solvent extracts. While the solvent extracts may not remain in the finished product, it's very hard to be sure. So you may want to read the label carefully if you purchase this type of product to verify it wasn't produced with solvents.

Hydrogenated Coconut Oil: As far as refined coconut oils go you want to stay away from these for any type of internal consumption. The small portion of unsaturated fatty acids are hydrogenated, which creates some trans fats and keeps the coconut oil solid at higher temperatures. Research at this time doesn't show this type of coconut oil being used in the edible market in the US. If this were to be used in the edible market it would most likely be used in candies in tropical regions of the world. RBD coconut oil will remain a solid up to 76 degrees Fahrenheit. In most tropical regions the temperatures run higher than that most of the time. So to keep it from melting it's hydrogenated before using it in margarines, candies, etc.

Liquid Coconut Oil: This is a relatively new product that showed up in 2013. The selling point was that it would stay liquid even when refrigerated. However, this is not a new product. This is actually fractionated coconut oil, an oil that has had the lauric acid processed out of it.

Some call it "MCT oil" or medium-chain triglyceride oil. Triglyceride is another term for fatty acids. In the past this was used in skin care products and now some are selling it as a dietary supplement that is edible.

MCT oil is actually a byproduct of the lauric acid industry. The lauric acid is a strong antimicrobial which makes it a great preservative commercially. It is a saturated fatty acid and comprises almost 50% of coconut oil. When you take it out of the coconut oil you end up with a lower melting point. So just know that when you see this product out in the marketplace it is highly refined and missing the all-important lauric acid.

So what about "<u>virgin coconut oils</u>"? Are they all the same?

All virgin coconut oils should start with fresh coconut, not copra. At this time though, there is no certifying body to make sure this is really true. In reality, anyone can label their product as "virgin" if they are of low integrity. Buying from a reputable company is always your best bet.

Extra Virgin Coconut Oil: How is that different from virgin coconut oil? It isn't. It's just a term used in marketing. There is no real difference between "extra virgin" and "virgin" coconut oil.

There are two broad categories of production that virgin coconut oils fall into.

1) Pressing the virgin coconut oil out of the dried coconut. First the white meat of the coconut is dried. Then at some point later on, that dried coconut meat is pressed and the oil extracted. By drying the coconut meat first it's easier to mass produce it. This is the most common way of producing virgin coconut oil. Since it starts with the actual coconut it is a much higher quality than oils starting with copra, even though it is mass produced.

2) The second process used to produce virgin coconut oil is known as "wet-milling". Here the oil is pressed out of fresh coconut meat, so the coconut meat is not dried before the oil is extracted. To do this the coconut milk is first pressed out of the coconut meat and then the oil is separated from the coconut milk. To separate out the coconut oil from the coconut milk the following methods are commonly used: refrigeration, enzymes, boiling, mechanical centrifuge and fermentation.

Research has found that virgin coconut oils produced by wet-milling contain a much higher percentage of antioxidants than those coconut oils produced by pressing dried coconut meat.

A number of studies have shown that the fermentation process of wet-milling produces a virgin coconut oil with highest number of antioxidants. This method has been used in coconut producing countries for centuries by the indigenous populations. It is a very simple process they still use in their kitchens today for personal consumption.

In the fermentation process freshly grated coconut meat is used to produce a coconut milk emulsion. That coconut milk emulsion is then allowed to sit overnight. During that period of time the heavier water sinks to the bottom and a clear layer of coconut oil floats to the top along with some of the coconut meat solids. The layer of coconut oil then gets skimmed off the top and heated in a pan until the coconut meat solids fall to the bottom. Then the oil is filtered for even further separation of the oil and what is left of the coconut oil meat. This process is still used by indigenous cultures today.

There was a study done in 2011 in Sri Lanka by Professor Kapila Seneviratne at the University of Kelaniya. That study showed that the process of wet-milling produced the highest level of antioxidants in coconut oil. What was most interesting about the study was the statistics showing that high heat actually increased the levels of antioxidants in the coconut oil. Before that study it was thought that high heat was detrimental to the antioxidant levels in coconut oil, which is why many manufacturers put "cold pressed" on their labels and didn't use any heat in their extraction processes.

This is a quote directly from the Sunday Times of Sri Lanka:

"More surprises awaited the research team. The general impression is that cooking at high temperatures would degrade the quality of the oil. However, it is not applicable since coconut oil is thermally stable, it is learnt. "Fortunately, most of the phenolic anti-oxidants present in coconut oil are also thermally highly stable," he pointed out, explaining that the reason for a greater composition of anti-oxidants is that simmering for a long time at a high temperature dissolved more anti-oxidants into the oil." (Published in The Sunday Times of Sri Lanka,

October 16, 2011 – "Coconut Oil: It's good for you after all," by Kumudini Hettiarachchi and Shaveen Jeewandara)

That was not the only study done on the effect of heat on antioxidant levels in virgin coconut oil. Another study was done in India in 2013 and published in the *Food Science and Biotechnology* journal. This study compared "cold extracted virgin coconut oil" (CEVCO) with "hot extracted virgin coconut oil" (HEVCO) and standard refined coconut oil (CCO). These were the results from their testing: *"antioxidant activity in the HEVCO group was 80-98%, 65-70% in CEVCO, and 34-45% in CCO."*

The conclusion of the above study was that coconut oils produced by wet-milling without heat contained lower levels of antioxidants than wet-milled coconut oils produced using heat.

The other consideration regarding coconut oils is whether or not to choose organic. This is a very costly process for growers and does supposedly guarantee no pesticides are used. At this time, I have found no GMO varieties of coconut to be out there. And very few pesticides are used by coconut growers. Coconuts grow very high up at the tops of the coconut trees so they are not sprayed, but that doesn't mean their roots may not absorb some type chemical or that a pesticide couldn't be injected directly into the sap of the tree.

Sensitivity Test: You should also always test a small amount of the coconut oil on your skin to make sure you have no sensitivities to it. If that comes out clear, then try a very small amount in your mouth to make sure that you are not allergic before you begin using coconut oil.

Now you know what kind of coconut oil to look for and eat and what kind to avoid. You've also learned how indigenous cultures make their own coconut oil using the fermentation method.

How do we turn off the "hunger monster" while burning off the fat? That's up next.

Coconut Oil in Weight Loss and Burning Fat

It's time now to find out how we can use coconut oil to feel full and eat less and just how coconut oil helps to burn off the pounds.

Almost everyone today is concerned about their weight. It has become a norm within our societies. This makes sense since our weight has an overall effect on our general health, either positive or negative. If we're overweight our organs have to work harder, thus wearing out faster and sooner. So keeping our weight at optimum level is greatly encouraged for good health.

One particular trend is to take supplements to improve health. While this is definitely worthwhile and at times advantageous, it can get out of control. We end up taking one supplement, then another, then another. And before we know it, we're taking handfuls of pills without remembering why we were taking what, all in an effort to improve our health and control our weight. Whatever happened to getting the nutrition we need through the foods we eat? Many of us have forgotten the importance of eating healthily.

One of the reasons coconut oil is so effective in weight loss goals is because it is nutrient and antioxidant dense. It has the effect of boosting your energy and suppressing your appetite at the same time. Many people have used it successfully for both of these reasons.

People who have switched to coconut oil have noticed weight loss, extra energy and fewer digestive disorders. Remember, coconut oil is quickly absorbed by the body and converted to energy by the liver. Many who take coconut oil are also less prone to falling ill because it has antioxidant and antibacterial properties which boost the immune system.

There are 3 main ways that virgin coconut oil helps you with weight loss:

1) Helps to decrease belly fat. This is a number one complaint for men and women as it seems to be one of the most stubborn fat areas. This area is targeted by the fat burning process brought on by virgin coconut oil.

2) Increases metabolism and helps your body to burn calories all day and all night. Even though it will boost the rate at which you're burning calories, you should still try to exercise. There's no substitute for moving and stretching the body. We weren't built to be couch potatoes!

3) Control blood sugar levels. This one is very important. Stabilizing blood sugar levels affects everything in the body. Sugar levels have a direct impact on weight loss and are directly responsible for the energy you experience during the day. Stable blood sugar levels help you to maintain your focus and your energy. You need both.

How Does Coconut Oil Burn Fat?

What makes it different from other oils? The secret is in the medium-chain fatty acids in virgin coconut oil.

Dr. Mercola cites the study of Dr. Mary Enig and Sally Fallon's explanation of the different types of fats and how they work differently in the body. Medium chain fatty acids are used differently than other body fats. They're used more like carbohydrates.

In the body medium-chain fatty acids are not freely circulating in the blood and they don't get stored in the tissue and added to body weight like other fats. They go directly to the liver and are converted to energy. An example of a large-chain fatty acid would be a steak. They are not metabolized by the liver and go to fat gain.

Be sure you're keeping your daily diet balanced. You're adding virgin coconut oil into a diet that should be made up of the correct portions of fiber, vitamins, minerals, fats, water, proteins and carbohydrates. This ensures you're getting everything you need for optimum metabolism and helps keeps you from feeling hungry and eating extra calories.

Do remember that even though virgin coconut oil has many benefits and features, it is an oil and high in fat, even though it is the good fat. So don't go overboard. The recommendation is to substitute virgin coconut oil for olive oil for weight loss. They both have about the same calories and fat: 119 calories and 13 grams of fat per tablespoon. The major difference is their liquidity: coconut oil is a solid at room temperature so has to be melted, whereas olive oil is already in a liquid state.

Coconut Oil as an Appetite Deterrent:

A teaspoon of coconut oil in hot tea or melted on the tongue can prove to be very effective at dealing with the munchies and an over-active appetite. Try this anytime you're looking for a quick bite or about 20 minutes before you eat and you'll likely find you eat less and are satisfied more quickly.

Taking coconut oil about 20 minutes before you eat goes a long way toward controlling hunger and cravings. You will feel satiated and be less prone to weight gain because the body doesn't see a need to store fats since it has a readily available supply of energy. This means consuming coconut oil will help prevent unnecessary weight gain. Coconut oil also boosts your metabolic rate and burns up to 3 times more calories.

While you can scoop coconut oil out and eat it solid, it goes down easier if you dissolve it into a favorite tea or cup of hot water first. My favorite is to add it to a cup of hot tea before meals. It makes me feel full so I eat smaller portions.

You can also dissolve it in hot water and add a few drops of herbal bitters, the kind used for digestion that can be purchased at the health food store. If you have a highly sensitive stomach, this is a good way to cut down on any queasiness you may feel when first starting to get used to taking coconut oil.

You've learned a lot so far. You just learned how virgin coconut oil helps you lose weight and how to use it to deter the appetite so you feel full, eat less and satisfy the body's needs.

The next thing we're delving into is the ugly secret of the hydrogenated oils as they get processed in the body. Once you learn this you'll find yourself avoiding them and automatically helping yourself shed the pounds.

Obesity, High Cholesterol and Hydrogenated Oils

Let's find out more specifics about these hydrogenated oils. What happens inside the body that makes us fat and what can we do to help ourselves avoid that?

High cholesterol levels and obesity have become so common place that just about everybody knows somebody who is either obese or has high cholesterol levels; in most cases, both. Consuming virgin coconut oil will naturally decrease the bad cholesterol levels and naturally restore the balance in your body. Your low-density lipoprotein (LDL) levels will be low and your good cholesterol levels will be high.

One of the problems we face in this country is the epidemic of obesity. The Journal of the American Medical Association states than nearly 1/3 of adults and 17% of youth in the United States are obese. And these statistics continue to rise.

But why? What has made obesity an epidemic? And why are there more people with high cholesterol than ever before?

There is one silent culprit that most people are unaware of. It is the toxic hydrogenated vegetable oils that are sold in stores and supermarkets all over the world. The oil manufacturing companies have created an image that portrays these vegetable oils as healthy, wholesome and beneficial. The stark reality is the opposite is true.

Just what is a hydrogenated oil and what makes it such a problem for the human body? Hydrogenated oils started out as oils that are actually good for you in their natural state. Those oils don't have a long shelf life so manufacturers put them through a chemical process to change that. The healthy oils are heated anywhere from 500 to 1000 degrees under several atmospheres of pressure.

Then a catalyst is injected into the oil for several hours. This catalyst is usually a metal like aluminum, nickel or platinum. As these metals are absorbed into the oil they change on a molecular level. So now the oil that was liquid at room temperature is either a solid or a semi-solid oil. This creates either fully hydrogenated oils or partially hydrogenated oils.

Unfortunately, these oils are now closer to cellulose and plastic than oil. Chemically, hydrogenated oil is only one molecule away from being classified as a plastic. The manufacturing companies love hydrogenated oils due to their ability to act as a preservative since all the enzymatic activity in the oil has been neutralized. So like plastics, they can last for years and not break down. If un-hydrogenated oils were used in foods, they would go bad very quickly and that would increase the cost to the manufacturer.

Your body is now trying to digest something that it never really can due to the plastic-like nature of hydrogenated oils; it just doesn't absorb since it's a foreign substance. Foreign substances cause false immune responses in the body which now strains the immune system and decreases the body's overall immunity.

Your body will continue to send more digestive acids/enzymes to the stomach to try and digest the plastic like oils. This in turn raises the temperature in the stomach causing a myriad of other health issues as well.

When you consume these hydrogenated oils your blood becomes thicker and more viscous just like the oil you're eating, which means your heart is working harder to move the thicker blood throughout your body. And it doesn't take a lot of time for this phenomenon to happen. Some studies show that negative side effects can occur within minutes of consuming foods containing hydrogenated oils. This is one of the ways that hydrogenated oils are contributing the high blood pressure so many people are experiencing.

Blood that has been made thicker by the hydrogenated oils is also stickier, so it lodges and gets stuck in arteries much easier and contributes more readily to arterial plaque. There are studies that show that these oils actually scar the internal walls of the arteries. This is from the nickel used in the hydrogenation process. When this happens the body reacts to try to protect itself by producing cholesterol to heal the scarred artery walls; so now there is plaque build-up on the arterial walls.

The more these hydrogenated oils are consumed, the worse it gets. By continually scarring the arterial walls the openings in the arteries slowly shrink giving less passageway for blood to move through. The heart is working even harder now to pump the necessary blood through, wearing it down faster.

The brain can now become affected. The heart has a harder time pumping the thicker blood through arteries that now have smaller openings, so less is reaching the brain. This slowing of the micro circulation of blood through the brain can contribute to muddled thinking and ailments like ADHD, Parkinson's, Alzheimer's, etc. As you may or may not know, aluminum has been linked to the onset of Alzheimer's disease. And aluminum is one of the metals sometimes used in the hydrogenation process.

Food is meant to break down quickly and digest itself with its enzymatic activity. Eating foods high in natural enzymes is good for you and consumes less energy from your own body. Examples of these types of foods are fresh vegetables, fruits and other types of raw foods such as nuts, seeds, etc.

The more dead food you consume the more your body has to create its own enzymes and use up its energy during digestion. This puts a huge strain on your internal organs, especially your pancreas since its job is to create the enzymes you need to digest your food. Overworking the pancreas is one of the major causes of Type II Diabetes, which is basically pancreatic failure.

You just learned how to help your body function better by making the switch from hydrogenated oils and how that will help you lose weight and control cholesterol. But did you know that in the good fat in coconut oil there's a secret ingredient proven to even destroy a virus? We'll talk about that next.

Saturated Fat Truths and the Immune System

We're going to delve into some of the research now and find out where all this information on good fats is coming from. And you'll learn about the virus combating property you automatically get when you go with coconut oil.

Coconut oil had a bad reputation for years. That's all changed now as new more complete information has come to light. Virgin coconut oil has finally received a new breath of life with recent studies showing that even though it is high in saturated fat, it is very beneficial to the body and not detrimental like the other oils.

The big question here is where are the saturated fats coming from? Manufactured or naturally produced?

In the 1930s a dentist by the name of Dr. Weston Price traveled extensively through the South Pacific studying the local cultures and the dental and physical health of the indigenous populations. What he found was a diet high in coconut consumption with slim, trim healthy populations where heart disease was almost unheard of.

Then in 1981 a study was done of two Polynesian cultures. Coconut was the main caloric staple of both groups. The results of that study were published in the *American Journal of Clinical Nutrition* indicating both populations exhibited strong vascular health. There was no evidence of harmful effects whatsoever on these populations in spite of the naturally occurring high saturated fat intake.

This is what Dr. Mercola has to say in an article published on his website October 22, 2010:

"It may be surprising for you to realize that the naturally occurring saturated fat in coconut oil actually has some amazing health benefits, such as:

Promoting your heart health

Promoting weight loss, when needed

Supporting your immune system health

Supporting a healthy metabolism

Providing you with an immediate energy source

Keeping your skin healthy and youthful looking

Supporting the proper functioning of your thyroid gland

But how is this possible? Does coconut oil have some secret ingredients not found in other saturated fats? The answer is a resounding "yes." "

The secret ingredient Dr. Mercola refers to in his article is lauric acid. This amazing ingredient comprises 50% of the fat content in coconut oil. Why is lauric acid so important to us?

The body is an amazing chemical factory. It converts lauric acid to monolaurin. Monolaurin has the ability to destroy the lipid coating on viruses. It's that lipid coating on a virus that makes it so impermeable to many drugs and medicines aimed at destroying it. Examples of such viruses are measles, flu, herpes, etc. Coconut oil contains more lauric acid than any other substance we know of. For this one reason alone, you should be considering adding virgin coconut oil to your diet.

The other thing to know about the saturated fats in virgin coconut oil is that almost 2/3 of it is made up of medium-chain fatty acids (MCFAs), also called medium-chain triglycerides (MCTs). Coconut oil is the best natural source of these MCTs.

By contrast, most of your common seed and vegetable oils are made up of long-chain fatty acids (LCFAs) also known as long-chain triglycerides (LCTs). Which is better? Medium chain triglycerides found in virgin coconut oil or long-chain triglycerides found in seed and vegetable oils?

Here's what happens in the body with long-chain triglycerides:

They can be left in your arteries as cholesterol.

They put additional strain on your digestive system, liver and pancreas.

They require special enzymes to break down, making them more difficult to utilize and requiring extra energy from the body to digest.

For the most part they get stored in the body as fat.

This is in contrast to the medium-chain triglycerides found in virgin coconut oil which have the following effects:

Easily digested, requiring less energy and strain on the entire digestive tract.

They are sent directly to the liver where they are converted into energy instead of being stored elsewhere as far.

Rev up your metabolism and help you burn fat and lose weight.

Since they are a smaller molecule, they pass through the cell membranes easier, rather than needing special enzymes for the body to use them effectively.

You can easily see how much more beneficial the medium-chain triglycerides found in virgin coconut oil are and how much additional benefit the body receives from them vs. consuming long-chain triglycerides found in many seed and vegetable oils.

Now we've learned the differences between the different kinds of fats and how they either help us or hurt us. Let's keep going to the rest of the body and find out how we can revive our brain and help it to function better, too.

Coconut Oil, Alzheimer's and Brain Health

Many of you are going to consider this chapter one of the most important since it deals with our brain. Without our brain functioning properly we have no quality of life. In this chapter we find out how we can help revive this all-important organ that controls how the body functions.

Just What Is Alzheimer's Disease?

The brain is just like any other part of the body. It needs energy to work. The brain prefers glucose as its primary energy source. In Alzheimer's disease patients the brain is unable to process glucose and produce the energy it needs to function. As a result of not getting the energy it needs, that part of the brain fails to work properly.

The Role of Virgin Coconut Oil In Brain Health

The human body converts two types of food groups into energy: glucose and fat. When the body uses a fat to produce energy, we end up with something called a ketone. Ketones are an alternative fuel used by the body when glucose is in short supply. Another important source of ketone production comes from medium-chain triglycerides (MCTs). We know that virgin coconut oil is an extremely rich source of these MCTs.

The processing of MCTs produces the chemical ketone Beta-hydroxybutyrate. Ketones are not only an alternative fuel source for the body, they protect the neurons of the brain while providing the energy to the brain cells. There are studies that show ketones play a factor in repairing, restoring and renewing damaged neurons.

Clinical Studies of Virgin Coconut Oil In Brain Health

There have been several stories about the miracle cure coconut oil can provide for those suffering the symptoms of Alzheimer's disease. People who love a good panacea have jumped on the wagon, but most of the stories that "prove" how effective miracle cures are prove to be wishful thinking in the end. So what is the story with coconut oil? Is it really a cure for Alzheimer's, and does it boost your brain health? Here are some answers that have scientific evidence behind them.

In 2004 a study was published in the journal *Neurobiology of Aging*. It determined that the medium-chain triglycerides (MCTs) in coconut oil improved cognitive function among older adults with diminished cognitive and memory function and even Alzheimer's disease. In this study 20 individuals were randomly fed virgin coconut oil or placebos on different days. Some of the members of the Alzheimer's group showed improved scoring on a special Alzheimer's cognitive rating scale and all of them demonstrated improved paragraph recall shortly after taking each dose of coconut oil.

While this wasn't a long-term study, it did show immediate positive cognitive and memory function from single doses of coconut oil compared to a placebo.

Other studies have also been conducted. A recent study was completed (due to be published in the

Journal of Alzheimer's Disease) that looked at how coconut oil may help to alleviate the symptoms associated with cognitive issues caused by neurodegenerative diseases. These types of diseases include Parkinson's, Alzheimer's and age-related dementia.

The study examined anecdotal evidence only (stories sent in by people but not medically verified) and looked for a consistency in the reporting to determine whether or not there was cause to study coconut oil further as a treatment or preventative for disease-related decline. What the study found was an overwhelming evidential pattern of patient experience that suggests coconut oil will help with the symptoms of cognitive decline.

Here is the excerpt of what was published so far in the *Journal of Alzheimer's Disease*, Volume 39, Number 2, 2014, pages 227-232:

"Coconut Oil Attenuates the Effects of Amyloid-β on Cortical Neurons in vitro

Abstract: Dietary supplementation has been studied as an approach to ameliorating deficits associated with aging and neurodegeneration. We undertook this pilot study to investigate the effects of coconut oil supplementation directly on cortical neurons treated with amyloid-β (Aβ) peptide in vitro. Our results indicate that neuron survival in cultures co-treated with coconut oil and Aβ is rescued compared to cultures exposed only to Aβ. Coconut oil co-treatment also attenuates Aβ-induced mitochondrial alterations. The results of this pilot study provide a basis for further investigation of the effects of coconut oil, or its constituents, on neuronal survival focusing on mechanisms that may be involved."

The Aβ peptide is the main component of certain deposits found in the brains of patients with Alzheimer's disease and is believed to contribute to the disease.

A group of medical researchers at Memorial University of Newfoundland, St. John's, NL, Canada conducted a pilot study. The study was focused on coconut oil directly supplied to the cortical neurons treated with Aβ peptide in vitro.

In clinical trials the researchers found significant improvement in Alzheimer patients after 45 to 90 days of treatment with medium-chain triglycerides (MCTs). The participants of the study were given a daily dose of medium-chain triglycerides by adding it to their diets. This study led to another trial study for a drug called Axona. Axona is a trade name for an FDA-approved caprylidene medical food. But Axona was doing nothing more than delivering the same MCT levels to the patient as 6 tablespoons of coconut oil a day.

What the researchers wanted to do in that study was find out if virgin coconut oil was beneficial for neurodegenerative issues using a cell model. They used live rat neurons and exposed them to various combinations of Aβ peptide and coconut oil. The result was that Aβ peptide reduced neuron survival and coconut oil protected against this Aβ peptide-induced reduction in survival time. The researchers found that not only did the peptides decrease on the affected neurons with treatment, but the damage done to the mitochondria appeared to start reversing.

The researchers noted that Aβ-cultured neurons that had been treated with coconut oil had a "healthier" appearance, and that coconut oil "rescued" Aβ-treated neurons from mitochondrial damage caused by toxicity. An additional observation was that coconut oil prevented Aβ-induced changes in the circuitry and size of mitochondria.

Why is this significant? In Alzheimer's patient's mitochondria function of the brain is often compromised. The main function of mitochondria is to take in nutrients from the cell, break them down, and turn that into energy. That energy then allows the cell to carry out its normal functioning. In this case we're talking about the cells of the brain.

MCT, Ketones and Crossing the Brain Barrier

One of the reasons that coconut is credited with being able to affect and repair the damage done by the peptides in neurodegenerative diseases is that the MCTs provide the brain with more of what it needs to resist damage. Another aspect that researchers are investigating is the properties of the ketones that coconut oil can provide for the body, and its ability to cross the brain barrier.

We learned earlier that ketones are what the body uses as a reserve fuel for all of its functioning. The ketones and MCTs provided by coconut oil are proven to cross the brain barrier (the barrier membrane that protects the brain). This makes it one of the few "supplements" or "superfoods" that are truly effective. While other sources can be found for MCT and ketones, very few are capable of crossing that barrier to actually help your brain. This may also explain why the addition of coconut oil to your daily diet can improve overall focus and memory and provide energy.

One other effect of coconut oil on the brain that was noticed during all of these studies is that it also has an anti-convulsant property. Coconut oil is looking very likely to live up to all the stories about it on the Internet. Unlike other natural panaceas touted as cure-alls, coconut oil is starting to have the evidence-based studies to support its claims.

You just learned about brain research, where to find more of it in more detail and how by adding virgin coconut oil to your diet you're reviving your brain at the same time.

We need to know how much coconut oil to take and for what situations. That's next.

How Much Coconut Oil Should I Take

Now let's answer the big question: How much is safe for me to take to get the results I want? Let's find out.

How much you take will depend on what you're taking it for, i.e., weight loss and general health or brain issues such as Alzheimer's.

Dosage for Weight Loss and General Health

There are no set standards for the consumption of virgin coconut oil. I've listed three sources and their consumption guidelines below. You'll need to read through them and decide what is best for you.

Dr. Oz recommends 30 milliliters or about 2 tablespoons a day. He bases his recommendation on a study done in 2009. In that study women who ate 30 milliliters of coconut oil a day for 12 weeks not only did not gain more weight, but had lower amounts of abdominal fat; fat that is the hardest to lose and contributes to heart problems.

This is where you can find that study and the clinical details:

http://www.ncbi.nlm.nih.gov/pubmed/19437058

Another source I found uses the following guidelines for those trying to lose weight. The weight listed is for your current weight:

90 to 100 pounds:

1 tablespoon before each meal 3 times a day

131 lbs to 180 pounds:

1.5 tablespoons before each meal 3 times a day

181 lbs and up:

2 tablespoons before each meal 3 times a day

And the American Heart Association makes its recommendation based on the number of calories you consume a day. They suggest limiting your daily intake of saturated fats to 5-6% of your daily caloric intake. They give this example: If you eat 2000 calories a day, less than 120 calories (or 13 grams) should come from saturated fats.

In coconut oil there are 117 calories in 1 tablespoon or 13.6 grams of fat. So their recommendation would be 1 tablespoon of coconut oil per day.

Whichever source you choose to follow will be up to you and your own research. As always, consulting your health professional is advised when changing dietary regimens.

There are two ways to take virgin coconut oil: in drink and food or directly into the mouth.

You can put virgin coconut oil directly into your mouth and let it melt there. But that may be a bit strong for many. For some, coconut oil is an acquired taste. It has a distinctive flavor and while some will take to it immediately, others need to adjust more slowly.

My suggestion is to start slowly, especially if you're consuming it directly without melting it into tea or food. Use a small amount like 1/8 to 1/4 teaspoon to start and let it melt in your mouth and see how you do. You can then increase to the higher amounts suggested if you prefer to consume it raw and directly instead of added to foods.

Gradual is better to make sure you don't end up queasy because you downed a tablespoon of coconut oil on an empty stomach. I've never had a problem, but I always melt mine in food or tea.

The second way to consume virgin coconut oil is in food and drink.

Let's face it, not everyone is going to like eating raw coconut oil. In fact, I'm guessing that will work for very few people, which is fine. There are all kinds of ways to utilize the recommended dosage without ingesting it a la carte. You'll get just as much benefit and will enjoy the taste by mixing it in with foods you already eat.

Coconut oil mixed in with a little honey and spread on toast is so yummy. And you can use the same mixture for sandwiches like peanut butter and jelly. Great unique flavor and it's so good for you.

Take a tablespoon and mix it in with steamed vegetables or rice. The heat will melt it quickly. Just stir it in.

It makes a very good salad dressing when mixed with a little lemon juice. Just melt the oil first. Or add it to your favorite salad dressing and mix it in that way.

One of my friends puts hers in her morning smoothie. It blends super easy and just becomes a part of the drink. You can do the same thing with shakes and yogurts.

My favorite way is to use about 1/8 teaspoon of coconut oil in hot tea. It sweetens the tea and gives it a rich consistency.

Always remember that coconut oil has calories in it, so keep that in mind and substitute coconut oil for other oils that you would normally consume.

Dosage For Brain Related Issues

It's important to keep in mind that improved memory from coconut oil is temporary and only last about 8 hours, which is why continued use of the product is required to keep the improvements. However, those same improvements happen almost immediately after consuming the coconut oil. Remember, coconut oil is processed in the liver and directly converted into energy and fuel.

I found these suggested guidelines at MySeniorSource.com regarding help for memory loss. (http://myseniorsource.com/topics/memory-care/how-coconut-oil-may-help-with-memory-loss)

Week One: One Tablespoon two times per day

Week Two: One Tablespoon three times per day

Ongoing: One Tablespoon four times per day

They make this notation: "You may take upwards of 6-8 tablespoons per day, but anything higher may result in loose stools. You may also increase to 2 tablespoons 3 times per day if it's difficult to remember a dose between meals."

For most people it's easier to consume the coconut oil with meals. You can use the same methods discussed earlier in this chapter.

Please remember these are suggested guidelines only, and what works for your body is individual and must be taken into consideration.

You just learned how much virgin coconut oil to take and how often to start changing your body and your life. And you learned the two different ways you can introduce it into your diet.

What about our skin? Rashes break out all the time and often we don't even know why. We just know we need something to help us deal with it. Next we're going to learn something we can do about it.

Can Coconut Oil Benefit Eczema?

Learning how to help our skin is one of the best things we can do. This next chapter will tell us how.

Skin issues are one of the major up-and-coming problems nowadays. More and more people are dealing with dry, itchy patches of skin out of nowhere. Sometimes the skin is scaly, dry, red, etc. These inflammatory conditions of the skin are commonly known as eczema and you can find a myriad of treatments available.

So what causes eczema? There can be any number of reasons for these skin conditions to crop up and without knowing what is causing yours, it can be difficult to treat and get rid of.

Sometimes eczema is due to contact with chemicals used in cosmetics, laundry products, latex, etc. Sometimes you just don't know where it's coming from. Consulting a dermatologist who can try to diagnose is always an option. A qualified skin doctor will often prescribe medical hydrators to help clear it.

We have an amazing immune system and the body will work tirelessly to try to overcome the inflammation on its own, but this can take time and make you extremely uncomfortable while waiting. And there is always the side effect of scarring that can occur from eczema, which is why so many people seek special treatment to deal with this.

Thousands of people have turned to virgin coconut oil to help relieve the symptoms of eczema. Coconut oil applied topically will often stop the itching and flaking. And this is in conjunction with avoiding the things that have caused the eczema to occur. Some find this even more effective if used in conjunction with the hydrators prescribed by their doctors.

One main way to use the coconut oil is to apply it directly to the skin and put a loose bandage over it. However, it's important to remember that the skin requires sunlight and fresh air, so you'll want to make sure you give the affected area those considerations as well.

The most important thing to remember is you only want to use virgin coconut oil. No processed coconut oil will do. Be sure it has no added perfumes or chemicals.

Using virgin coconut oil for eczema is getting good reviews from individuals and clinical studies. It will kill off microbial infections and moisturize at the same time, making it a great topical for damaged skin.

But first you must find out if you're going to be one of the few who will have an allergic reaction. Apply a little to a small area of skin and wait for 30 minutes. If after that period of time you have no adverse reactions, apply to larger areas.

You just learned how to do a patch test to make sure you're not sensitive. And you learned how to use coconut oil to help with those dry itchy patches. Up next we want to learn about helping to save our hair. What can we do to make our hair lustrous, decrease breakage and help it to regrow?

Coconut Oil For Hair

In this chapter you'll learn how to save yourself money by using coconut oil instead of expensive chemical-laden products. And you'll learn how to deal with dandruff, breakage and thinning hair, too.

One of the great things about using coconut oil on your hair is the complete absence of all the chemicals you so commonly find in most hair care products on the store shelves today.

An article was published in *Journal of Cosmetic Science* about coconut oil. It showed that coconut oil out-performed mineral oil and sunflower oil, and was the only oil they found that reduced protein loss. Protein loss is what leads to damaged dry hair that breaks.

As you know, coconut oil is high in lauric acid. Lauric acid has a low molecular weight. This makes it able to penetrate the hair shaft pulling the vitamins, minerals and medium-chain fatty acids found in coconut oil along with it. This nourishes and strengthens the hair and helps to control the damage from over-brushing and combing.

Coconut oil is a great hair conditioner and can be used as a leave-in conditioner, an intensive overnight conditioner, or concentrated 2-hour conditioner. If you're going to be using coconut oil as a leave-in conditioner you need to find the right amount for your hair. A little goes a long way and this is not the time to go overboard in your application.

How to use coconut oil as a leave-in conditioner:

Coconut oil is a great leave-in conditioner for the hair and has an SPF of 8, so will help to protect your hair from sun damage.

The amount of coconut oil you use will depend on the amount of hair you have. Use this as a beginning guideline:

Shorter Hair: Start with 1/4 teaspoon

Thicker, Longer Hair: Increase amount used up to 1/2 tablespoon

Thin Hair: Go sparingly, maybe only 1/8 teaspoon to start out in the beginning.

Put the coconut oil in the palms of your hands and let it warm and melt. Then smooth evenly throughout the hair and style normally. Focus on applying to the shaft and ends of the hair, not the root.

If you have thin hair, then go lightly with this process. Oil can weigh thin hair down if you use too much.

To use coconut oil as an intensive conditioner:

Coconut oil is a great restorative and intensive conditioner. Deep conditioning at-least once a month helps to restore the vitality to damaged hair from heat styling, washing and various hair care products.

First shampoo hair as you usually would with a gentle shampoo.

Then use this guideline and adjust as needed:

For short hair: 1 teaspoon

For shoulder length hair: 2 teaspoons

For long hair: 1 tablespoon

Warm the oil between the palms of your hands and let it melt. Apply the coconut oil to the hair shafts and ends, and then rub into the scalp. Take a shower cap and cover the hair. At this point leave the coconut oil in the hair for 1 or 2 hours or overnight, whichever is your preference. When you've reached the designated time limit wash your hair with a gentle shampoo and style as you normally would.

What about the frizzies and split ends?

Frizzy, fly-away hair is a problem for many people, especially in the winter when there is less moisture in the air. If your hair is overly dry and lacking in the normal essential oils, you can also get the frizzies.

Rub a dab of coconut oil (1/4 teaspoon to 1 teaspoon usually depending on how much hair you have) between your hands and let it melt. Then lightly run your fingers through to the ends of your hair. Give yourself a few extra minutes of blow drying time since it will take a little longer with the oil in your hair, but the results are worth it when you see how shiny and soft your hair is. This also helps deal with split ends as well.

Is dandruff a concern for you?

Coconut oil has been used for decades by people in the know when it comes to dealing with dandruff. The flaky, itchy scalp known as dandruff is often caused by sensitive skin that doesn't do well with the chemicals found in many hair care products, as well as dry skin and common fungal infections such as Malassezia. Malessezia is a type of fungi that grows on sebaceous areas of the body such as the scalp, face and upper trunk.

Coconut oil consists of medium-chain fatty acids that contain lauric acid and capric acid. Both of these acids have strong antimicrobial, antifungal and antiviral properties. These properties will hone in on the fungus and any other virus and bacteria on the scalp and help to kill them.

There are essential oils that are very effective in fighting dandruff, especially when mixed in with coconut oil. Before using any of these essential oils be sure you are not allergic or sensitive to them. You only need one of the oils mentioned, so if you find you're sensitive to one of them just don't use it.

Here are some oils to consider: Tea Tree Oil, Lavender, Thyme and Wintergreen

To treat dandruff, try this:

Put 5 drops of one of the oils listed above into 2 teaspoons of coconut oil and mix together thoroughly. Then massage that mixture directly into your scalp and cover your head with a shower cap for 20-30 minutes. To make it more intensive, add heat by sitting in the sun or under a hair dryer on the lowest setting.

After the allotted time, remove the shower cap and wash your hair as you usually would. Use this procedure 2 to 3 times a week to continue controlling the dandruff.

Are you worried about thinning hair?

One of the safest and least expensive aids to re-growing hair is coconut oil. Due to the lauric acid, Vitamin E, Vitamin K and other essential nutrients in coconut oil it can help to grow your hair thicker and longer.

Most of us have experienced stress that has damaged our hair in some way. Maintaining a healthy diet is one way to help keep hair healthy. Consuming foods high in Omega-3 fats will help to nourish hair from the inside out. Flaxseed and flaxseed oil, chia seeds, salmon and nuts are just a few of the foods you can eat to increase your levels of Omega-3s.

Know that most prescription hair growth products only work for 50% of the people that try them and require continued use. Before going that route, try changing your diet and add coconut oil use to your hair care regimen.

How to use coconut oil for hair growth:

Massage increases circulation. When you massage your scalp you're improving the oxygen and blood percentages that reach the hair roots and follicles. If you add coconut oil to the massage, you'll be massaging the nutrients and lauric acid of the coconut oil into your scalp and hair.

Put about 1 teaspoon of coconut oil into the palm of your hands, let it melt, and then massage directly into the scalp for 10 minutes. Now place a shower cap on your head or wrap your scalp with plastic wrap to hold in the heat of the body coming up through the scalp. This will warm the hair and oil you've just rubbed in and deepen the treatment. You can leave this on for 20-30 minutes if you'd like, then shampoo as you normally would.

Do this 3 or 4 times a week and you'll be improving the growth of your hair and conditioning your scalp at the same time.

Rosemary oil is an essential oil that is known to increase new hair growth that can be added to this regimen for hair growth if you want. First make sure you're not allergic or sensitive to the rosemary oil. If not, then add 3 or 4 drops of rosemary essential oil to the teaspoon of coconut oil and use that mixture to massage the scalp per the same procedure discussed above. People have reported great results by adding this essential oil to the treatment.

These treatments work well for over-treated hair also, as well as losing too much hair from washing and brushing.

You learned so many things from this chapter: How to save money on hair care products while getting amazing results, getting rid of dandruff and secrets to help your hair grow long and strong.

But what about the rest of our body: specifically, our gums and teeth? Is there also an inexpensive, healthy way to improve oral and dental health, too? Yes! We find that out next.

What Is Oil Pulling and How Does It Help Oral Health?

Gums and teeth are a primary concern for all of us and now we're going to learn what we can do at home for just pennies to help both.

Most people have never heard of oil pulling. The process originated in India where it has been practiced for the last 3000 years and is a part of their folk medicine and Ayurvedic traditions.

Over the past few years more and more research has been done on the benefits of oil pulling and in natural health circles it's become quite popular. Unlike some home remedies, oil pulling has proven scientific benefits. While the majority of the studies are focused on oral health, there have been benefits in relieving sinus congestion noted as well.

Before you make up your mind one way or the other about this unusual little process, let's review some of the benefits that have been proven as well as anecdotal benefits that have been reported, but not necessarily studied as yet.

It should be noted that a variety of oils can be used for oil pulling. Since sesame oil is easily obtained and a staple in India, the studies below were conducted using it. Virgin coconut oil contains lauric acid a powerful antiviral and antibacterial, making it extremely popular to use in oil pulling in other world cultures.

In 2009 a study published in the *Indian Journal of Dental Research* found that when compared with mouthwash, oil pulling reduced plaque, modified gingival scores and lowered microorganisms in the plaque of 20 adolescent boys with plaque-induced gingivitis.

In 2014 in the *Journal of Clinical and Diagnostic Research* a study was published using 60 students at Maharani College. The results of that study showed that oil pulling helped to reduce the malodor and oral microbes as much as a chlorhexidine treatment. And in 2011 the *Journal of the Indian Society of Pedodontics and Preventive Dentistry* found oil pulling as effective as chlorhexidine for treating bad breath.

Many people have had the following effects of oil pulling:

- Brighten appearance of teeth
- Improved tooth, gum and jaw health
- Relief from congested sinuses
- Body detoxification

Photos of teeth being whitened using oil pulling can be found on the Internet, along with a number of personal stories from people trying the process. Some users of oil pulling even say it prevents cavities since you're pulling the bacteria from the mouth. I've not found a study to confirm that yet.

The methods are very simple, but it does take time and it does produce better and better results the longer you do it. The belief is that since coconut oil is antibacterial and antiviral by nature, it will kill the harmful bacteria in your mouth and also extract any impurities from your body.

For this method you will need:

1 teaspoon of solid coconut oil to start; you can work your way up to 1 tablespoon as time progresses if you choose.

1 glass of warm water

Oil Pulling Procedure:

Swish ½ of the glass of warm water around in your mouth then spit it out. This will dislodge any debris stuck between the teeth.

Put the teaspoon of coconut oil in your mouth. Let it warm and melt.

Now swish it around somewhat vigorously. You can either swish for 10 to 20 minutes or do 2 sessions of 4 minutes each, depending on what works best for you. Be careful not to swallow any. It's now full of toxins you're pulling out of the oral cavity.

Spit out all of the coconut oil.

Rinse out your mouth with the remainder of the warm water and spit it out as well.

Wait about 20 minutes before brushing your teeth and drinking or eating anything.

There are two other traditional Ayurvedic methods that are also used: Kavala and Gandusa.

In the Kavala method you hold the coconut oil in your mouth for a couple minutes, swirl it around some, and then spit it out. This should only take 3-4 minutes and is repeated 2 to 4 times.

The Gandusa method is simpler. Just hold the coconut oil in your mouth 3-5 minutes and then spit it out. You don't need to swirl.

One of the biggest problems people have when first starting oil pulling is trying to do it too long. The taste can be strong in the beginning. Try the two shorter time frames mentioned above to begin with and see how you do with that. If that works for you, you can continue with those or go onto longer time periods, whatever you prefer.

Here are some tips for oil pulling many have found useful:

If you don't like the taste, add a drop of peppermint to the oil before your start.

To save time, you can do the oil pulling when in the shower. This makes the time go faster and it's less noticeable.

Don't start with too much oil. The saliva will build up in the mouth along with the coconut oil. If you end up with too much as you go along, just spit out the excess and continue.

Most research has found the morning before you eat to the best time to oil pull. Science finds it creates an easier environment for oral health.

Take before and after pictures. This is a cumulative process and to see the real results you need to give it 30 to 45 days of daily consistent use. If you take photos you won't just imagine something has happened, you'll be able to see it in front of you.

Oil pulling is said to prevent cavities, reduce plaque buildup and strengthen your gums. It's also said that the coconut oil will prevent many sicknesses from taking root in your body because of the antiviral and antibacterial nature of coconut oil.

Dentists have mentioned that oil pulling has no conclusive evidence that it works. Because of this, normal brushing and flossing should not be forgotten just because one does oil pulling. The best course of action will be to brush and floss daily and also spend a few minutes doing oil pulling. You can do both. Oil pulling is not a mutually exclusive activity.

Just like there are two sides to a coin, there is a side effect of coconut oil that you should be aware of. In most cases, the side effect occurs because people are too eager to see benefits and consume too much coconut oil too soon in order to accelerate the results.

If you consume too much coconut oil in a short space of time, you will most probably get diarrhea. This is a result of the medium-chain fatty acids making your stools soft and loose.

The best way to avoid all these side effects will be to consume just a teeny bit of coconut oil each day when you are starting out. The same applies for oil pulling. Over time as your body gets more accustomed to the coconut oil, you may slowly increase the amount. In this way, your body will adapt and get all the benefits that coconut oil has to offer.

You just learned an easy, inexpensive way to dramatically improve your gums and your teeth.

You also learned how that same process pulls toxins out that could have been harmful to your organs.

There are so many ways that coconut oil can save you money in the kitchen, in your beauty routines and more. We'll cover that next.

Coconut Oil Uses You May Not Know About

This chapter is going to teach you fun and helpful ways to use coconut oil you've probably never thought of.

Coconut oil is one of the most versatile products I've found. It is extremely beneficial to the body and your health and a great commodity to have around the house for so many things.

Here are several uses for coconut oil that I've found make life simpler. Incorporate some of these now to start developing new body-conscious health habits.

<u>Coconut Oil Uses in Cooking and in the Kitchen:</u>

Use it for cooking. It has a high smoke point and that makes it better than olive oil if you're baking or frying food. Try using it to replace your normal cooking oil such as olive oil (especially if you're trying to lose weight). Several cooking oils aren't meant to be used on high heat, but coconut oil can be used at any temperature range. The same thing applies to the non-stick sprays with all the chemicals and other ingredients. Skip those sprays and stay with the coconut oil. You'll also get a richer flavor.

Coconut oil is a great replacement for butter if you're trying to quit consuming dairy products. It's really good on toast. Just spoon and spread for creamy rich texture that's good for you.

Mix a little coconut oil in your drinks or food for an energy booster. The virgin coconut oil will boost your metabolism and help burn off the fat. The medium-chain triglycerides will help burn off the excess calories.

Want a great popcorn treat that's also butter and salt free? Use a skillet with a little virgin coconut oil to make your popcorn on the stove. You'll get a great flavor without the added calories and the oil can handle the high heat. If you really miss the oil directly on the popcorn, just melt a little virgin coconut oil and pour over the popcorn and stir it around. I like the taste much better and it's still rich and satisfying.

Sweet potato chips are all the rage now and so tasty with virgin coconut oil. Just slice the sweet potato into 1/8" thicknesses. Put the slices on a cookie sheet and then brush them with the coconut oil. Bake at 400 degrees for about 15 minutes, serve and eat. Yummy!

You can use virgin coconut oil to replace any oil you would normally use in your baking. Just replace the oil that is called for with the same amount of coconut oil. That's it! No other change to make.

Pan frying works the same way. Use coconut oil instead of any other oil you'd usually use. I love to do this with scrambled eggs. It's so much richer tasting and better for me. Or try it the next time you fry chicken and see what you think.

My friend loves to use virgin coconut oil when she makes a grilled cheese sandwich. She was a little skeptical at first, but now that's the only way she makes it!

Want to make that coffee sweet and even more of an energy boost? Add a teaspoon of virgin coconut oil. Works for tea, too!

For <u>salads</u> I melt a little virgin coconut oil and mix in a little lemon juice. This has become my favorite dressing and it's so inexpensive to make.

Need to <u>season a cast iron skillet</u>? Rub coconut oil on the inside of the pan after it's been cleaned.

<u>Coconut Oil Uses in Skin Care and Beauty Regimens</u>:

My main <u>moisturizer</u> is now virgin coconut oil. I just put a little dab on my fingers and rub them together. The warmth of the skin will melt it instantly, then apply to the skin. No expensive chemical-laden <u>facial creams</u> for me!

For <u>acne and problematic skin</u>, try using this homemade combination of baking soda and coconut oil. Baking soda is an amphoteric compound and can be used to correct the pH balance. Combined with the antibacterial properties of coconut oil, it becomes a great exfoliant for the skin, helping to polish off the dead skin layers and remove built-up debris in the pores.

Use a 2:1 ratio of coconut oil to baking soda for sensitive skin. You can use a 1:1 ratio if you want a more aggressive mixture. Mix the two together and apply to the skin, wet or dry. You can let it sit on the skin like a mask for a few minutes or gently wash it off with warm water in circular motions. The latter method will give you more of an exfoliation treatment. While you can store it if you make up more than one application's worth, it's best to make up only what you'll use in one application for sanitation's sake.

Shaving creams are now a thing of the past for me. I just use coconut oil. Not only am I missing out on all those chemicals, but it also won't dry out my skin like soaps.

Try using virgin coconut oil as a massage oil. It's great for hydrating the skin.

Use it for reducing the appearance of fine lines on the face. Again, it's super hydrating.

You can use coconut oil as a highlighter for your cheeks. Just do your makeup as you normally would, and then dab a little bit on cheekbones for a healthy natural glow that compliments any shade of makeup you're wearing.

Coconut oil is great for taking off makeup. I find it as effective as the store bought makeup remover. And it's completely natural, not filled with chemicals.

Many have found coconut oil does a great job in lightening age spots since it's full of antioxidants. Just apply virgin coconut oil to the skin, especially if you've just come back from being outside in the sun. Continue to apply until they fade away.

Stretch marks can be reduced by rubbing the coconut oil onto the skin. This is great for pregnant women and for those who've acquired the marks from rapid weight gain or loss.

Painful cracked skin on your heels? Coconut oil rubbed into dry cracking areas a few times a day will help the skin heal and become soft again.

I make my own facial scrubs using coconut oil. Use a tablespoon of sea salt or any other large crystal salt and 1/4 cup of virgin coconut oil. You can also add a few drops of your favorite essential oil like lavender or lemongrass. Stir and scrub. You'll have enough left over for additional uses, so be sure to store in an airtight jar. It's also a great exfoliant for those dry elbows and heels.

Love the facial scrub so much you want a body scrub, too? Add a tablespoon of sugar to 1/2 cup of coconut oil. Add your desired favorite essential oil if you want, stir and use. This also makes a great gift. Find a pretty jar, increase the recipe, seal the jar and tie it off with a bow when you're done and you've made someone very happy and saved money!

Deodorant can sometimes be a problem for sensitive skin. Homemade deodorant is simple to make using coconut oil. Just add some baking soda and apply. No harmful chemicals to irritate those delicate areas. Another recipe for homemade deodorant is to mix the coconut oil with arrowroot powder, baking soda, cornstarch and a scented oil such as lavender.

Dry chapped lips? I grab a cotton swab and use it straight out of the jar. It's so effective and easy.

Use coconut oil as an all-over skin moisturizer in the bath. You can either melt 1/4 cup of coconut oil and pour it into the bath or melt a little and apply to the skin after you bathe. Either way, it's wonderfully hydrating.

Gargle with a spoonful of coconut oil daily and it will help freshen your breath due it's anti-fungal and anti-bacterial properties.

Coconut oil is one of the best cuticle oils I've found. Rub it in at the base of the nail. It will also help your manicure last longer, too.

We all need to keep our <u>makeup brushes clean</u> and germ free. Washing them at least once a month is best. Try this recipe: mix two parts of your favorite soap and one-part coconut oil. Not only will your brushes be clean, the coconut will help to condition the bristles.

Great homemade <u>toothpaste</u> is simple to make. Use one-part coconut oil with one-part baking soda. Tastes great, whitens and saves money!

<u>Coconut Oil for Various Health Issues:</u>

How does virgin coconut oil help combat viruses and boost your immune system? The secret is in the lauric acid, a saturated fat that many people are now using for a number of different ailments.

According to webmd.com (webmd.com/vitamins-supplements/ingredientmono-1138-lauric%20acid.aspx?activeingredientid=1138&activeingredientname=lauric%20acid), lauric acid is used for treating viral infections, influenza, cold sores, the common flu, and different forms of herpes as well as a number of other maladies. To date, science doesn't know exactly how lauric acid works medically.

A regimen of daily coconut oil will do wonders for more than just weight loss.

Studies have shown that countries in Southeast Asia which use coconut oil do not have as many diseases as the Western nations. Obesity, diabetes, cholesterol, blood pressure, etc. are not as prevalent.

Make coconut oil a part of your diet and reap the rewards. It is one of the healthiest supplements on the planet and it's inexpensive. This is not a privilege that only the wealthy can afford. Coconut oil is very inexpensive and most people can afford it.

Keep reading for some ways to implement virgin coconut oil into your lifestyle right away.

That morning energy boost is easy to get with virgin coconut oil. Have a spoonful in the morning to get your metabolism up and running without the nervous jittery edge of a stimulant like coffee.

Control your appetite. Have a teaspoon of coconut oil about 20 minutes before a meal. You'll find you're less hungry, eat less and the pounds come off easier.

<u>Have an itchy rash</u>? Mix tea tree oil into virgin coconut oil. Tea tree oil is a potent anti-fungal and mixed with the coconut oil gives relief from burning and itching. Shower or clean the area, then apply the mixture. You can pat it dry once it has set if you want to.

You may need to apply daily until the rash disappears which may take weeks depending on your situation, so don't be impatient. Getting rid of the burn and itch is worth it. This works for bug bites, too. And as always, only use products you know you're not allergic to. Do the patch test if you have any doubt or concern.

<u>Yeast Infections</u>: Coconut oil has been laboratory proven to explode the nucleus of Candida yeast cells. It has also been shown to control irritation and reduce inflammation of the vaginal area.

Coconut oil is high in lauric, capric and caprylic acid, three ingredients that have antiviral, antimicrobial and anti-fungal properties. These target the bad bacteria while leaving the good bacteria untouched.

Caprylic acid will break down the cell membrane of yeast which stops it from replicating and destroys it.

The lauric acid will strengthen the body's immune system while giving it the support it needs to fight off the yeast fungus.

Coconut oil is an antioxidant and therefore an effective agent in destroying not only harmful yeast but a myriad of other types of excessive fungal growths in the body.

When coconut oil is applied to sensitive infected areas it forms a barrier against chafing and helps to quickly heal the irritated skin as it's natural antibacterial and antifungal properties kick in.

To use virgin coconut oil to help control yeast:

Use it in your diet as I've talked about throughout this book.

Also, apply a thin layer to the affected area once it's been cleaned and air dried. You'll want to do this application 2-3 times a day until the yeast infection is gone.

To use it as a douche, mix 3-4 tablespoons in 2 quarts of warm distilled water and repeat daily until the yeast infection has cleared. Or you can use a tampon dipped in virgin coconut oil in place of the douche.

Diaper rash symptoms can be soothed naturally with coconut oil, which means no harmful chemicals on baby's tender skin. And it hydrates and heals as it moisturizes.

Are allergies a problem for you? Here's a great little trick to try. Lightly rub some coconut oil on the inside of your nose and watch symptoms dissipate. Don't stuff it all the way up into the sinus cavities. Melt the coconut oil and dip your finger into it, then apply to the lower interior nasal areas.

Do you have poor circulation or do you always feel cold? The healthy fats and medium-chain triglycerides help relieve inflammation in the arteries. That then improves the blood flow in the body. Consume 2-3 tablespoons of virgin coconut oil daily to help combat the poor circulation that is making you feel cold. You can also rub the coconut oil onto the hands and legs daily to absorb it through the skin.

Cold Sores: Since coconut oil is antiviral it can also be applied topically to a cold sore to help heal it and keep it from cracking and bleeding. Be sure to use a cotton swab to get the coconut oil out of the jar onto the cold sore. You don't want to transmit the virus into the coconut oil in the jar.

<u>Diabetes:</u> The body sends the medium-chain fatty acids found in virgin coconut oil directly to the liver making it a great source of energy for the body. The really great thing about virgin coconut oil is that it does not produce an insulin spike in the bloodstream, which means coconut oil has the effect of a carbohydrate without any of the negative affects you get from eating high amounts of carbs long term. So to sum it up, with virgin coconut oil you get a fast acting energy source with no insulin spike.

Pregnenolone:

Another benefit of coconut oil is that it converts cholesterol into pregnenolone. Dr. Raymond Peat, a leading researcher in the field of hormones, shows that coconut products that are regularly added to a balanced diet will <u>lower cholesterol</u> levels to normal by converting them into pregnenolone. Pregnenolone is the precursor to many hormones in the body including progesterone. Dr. Peat has recommended that women with <u>hormone</u>

imbalances should increase their levels of pregnenolone.

Pregnenolone is one of the major factors that give coconut oil and coconut products their reputation as beautifying agents. Pregnenolone reduces bags under the eyes by promoting the contractions of muscle-like cells, improves circulation in the skin and restores sagging skin.

Pregnenolone also improves memory, protects the nerves from stress, and has anti-anxiety properties.

These are just some of the many uses and benefits of coconut oil. With a little imagination and some research on the Internet you can come up with even more. Since it's convenient and inexpensive, it's become one of my main "go-to" sources for everyday health improvement.

You learned a lot from this chapter, like how coconut oil helps with sagging skin, how to make popcorn yummy, and the anti-anxiety benefits you get from coconut oil use.

But how does coconut oil compare to olive oil? Should you still be using both or just coconut oil? We'll find out by reading the next chapter.

Should I Use Coconut Oil or Olive Oil?

This is where you'll learn about olive oil and what its benefits are as compared to coconut oil.

If I have to choose just one, which is better: Coconut oil or olive oil?

This seems to be a question that many people are asking. The answer is they are both good in their own ways and there is a time for each. Comparing the two is like comparing apples and oranges. You don't have to be exclusive and choose one over the other. It will depend on what type of oil you need for the intended application.

Here are some points to consider when deciding which oil to use for what occasion.

Two of the most popular diets we're hearing about right now are the Mediterranean diet and the Paleo diet. The Mediterranean diet uses a lot of extra virgin olive oil. The Paleo diet is a proponent of virgin coconut oil.

Since the Mediterranean diet emphasizes staying away from processed foods and the Paleo diet has you eating meats and foods that need to be cooked, they are utilizing different oils. Olive oil has a low smoke point and incurs oxidative damage at high heat. Coconut oil is more stable at higher temperatures and therefore healthier for cooking at the higher temperatures.

So, for cooking in high heat, coconut oil is better. For foods that require just a drizzle of oil, such as salads, etc. go with the olive oil.

The other thing to take into consideration is the number of calories you're consuming from fats. Yes, both coconut oil and olive are beneficial oils with a number of health benefits. They are also fats and should be utilized in moderation just like any other food.

Here are a couple of differences to consider, assuming you are eating 2000 calories a day. Coconut oil is made up of saturated fat and 2 tablespoons of virgin coconut oil will hit the daily limit of saturated fat for most people. Conversely, olive oil is mostly unsaturated fat and it takes 6 tablespoons to hit the daily limit of unsaturated fat in the same scenario.

In terms of grams of fat per tablespoon, both oils are the same at 14 grams per tablespoon.

As far as calorie count goes, in one tablespoon of virgin olive oil you will get 119 calories. In one tablespoon of virgin coconut oil you will get 116 calories. The calorie counts are almost the same.

Both oils have zero cholesterol.

One tablespoon of extra virgin olive oil has 1 gram of saturated fat. One tablespoon of virgin coconut oil has 12 grams of saturated fat.

The opposite is true of monunosaturated fat. One tablespoon of extra virgin olive oil has 9.8 grams and one tablespoon of coconut oil has 0.8 grams.

In polyunsaturated fat you'll get 1.4 grams in one tablespoon of extra virgin olive oil and .2 grams in one tablespoon of virgin coconut oil.

One big difference is, coconut oil will boost your metabolic rate and it has been shown that coconut oil burns three times more calories in the body. This is something that olive oil does not do. So, coconut oil has fat burning properties and is better for those trying to lose weight.

Another thing to consider is taste. Olive oil has a milder taste and most people are accustomed to the flavor. Coconut oil has a stronger flavor and some people may take some time getting used to it (which is why it's best to start off slowly in its use).

If you're having company for dinner you may want to use olive oil. Even though the benefits of coconut oil are clear, the taste could be too much for someone who has never used it. So on those occasions you may want to stick with the olive oil.

Antifungal, antibacterial and antimicrobial properties are another big plus for the use of virgin coconut oil. People with skin conditions find the use of virgin coconut oil highly beneficial in combating those issues and will apply the coconut oil topically along with eating the oil.

Consumption of virgin coconut oil is also of great benefit for those with digestive issues. These conditions have a tendency to diminish when coconut oil is eaten on a regular basis.

Both oils have a number of additional uses as well, such as massage, body moisturizers, etc.

As you can see, both oils are useful and healthy, and both should be utilized in the appropriate circumstances. One thing you'll want to do in almost every case is to discontinue the use of hydrogenated oils completely and use coconut oil and olive oil instead.

Read labels and know what you're getting. Often hydrogenated oils are being touted as natural and healthy, but careful examination of the label will show otherwise. You're better off staying with oil you know the true value of.

You just learned how beneficial both olive oil and coconut oil can be in the right circumstances. You also learned what the differences are so you know when it's appropriate to use which one.

Did you know there are other parts of the coconut that are also beneficial and nutritious? Coconut milk can also help you lose weight. Let's find out how it works next.

What Is Coconut Milk?

Here we'll find out what coconut milk is and what it is not. And we'll find out what type of coconut milk is best.

Coconut milk is actually made, not naturally grown. When you first open a coconut, the milky white substance that pours out of the center is coconut water, not coconut milk. To get coconut milk you have to blend the meat of the coconut with water.

It's the younger, less mature coconuts that have more water in them than meat. The longer a coconut grows, the more of the water is replaced by the white meat. Coconut water has a higher electrolyte content than coconut milk, which is higher in the good saturated fats. Like coconut oil, coconut milk can help to lower cholesterol levels and improve blood pressure.

Coconuts are quite nutritious. They are high in vitamins B5, B6, B1, E and C and good sources of the minerals calcium, magnesium, iron, selenium, sodium and phosphorous.

Full fat coconut milk is also high in calories. It's best to consume it in smaller servings than you would regular cow's milk or coconut water. For calorie's sake try staying with 1/4 to 1/2 cup at a time. You can either drink it straight, put it in smoothies, on cereal or experiment to see what venue works best for you.

Here are some nutrition facts on full fat coconut milk:

1/4 cup will yield 138 calories, 1/5 gram of protein, 2 grams of sugar and 14 grams of fat

Unlike cow's milk, coconut milk is lactose free making it an excellent choice for those that are lactose intolerant. It is also very popular with vegans where it is used as an alternative to dairy in baking, as well as smoothies, shakes and energy drinks. It is also quite popular in curry dishes.

What Is the Best Type of Coconut Milk?

In my opinion, the best coconut milk you can get is the coconut milk you make yourself from organic coconut. See the recipe I have included on making your own coconut milk in a later chapter in this book.

If you're not a do-it-yourself type, then use these guidelines to ensure you're getting the purest you can find.

Look for coconut milk that is organic if possible, has no added sugar or sweeteners and isn't pasteurized. Pasteurization can destroy vitamins and minerals. Avoid the sweeteners if you don't want to get hit with too much sugar. You can add sweeteners at home if it isn't sweet enough for you.

Try to find coconut milk that is "cold pressured," meaning minimum processing and heat exposure has been used to remove bacteria and preserve nutritional content.

Read the label carefully. You're looking for the primary ingredient to be 100% coconut milk and possibly coconut water. There are some companies that add guar gum to stabilize texture. Guar gum is a fiber from the seed of the guar plant. Some of its uses are: as a laxative, in the treatment of diarrhea, irritable bowel syndrome, obesity, diabetes, reducing cholesterol and prevention of hardening of the arteries. Guar gum is used industrially as a binding agent in tablets and thickener in creams and lotions.

Most people will have no problems with guar gum. But it does have side effects for some such as diarrhea, loose stools and increased gas. Make sure you read labels if you're someone with no tolerance for guar gum.

Now we know that there are different types of coconut milk, what to look for and what to avoid.

Let's find out about the health benefits coconut milk provides, including its effects on cholesterol. The next chapter will tell us.

What Health Benefits Does Coconut Milk Provide?

This chapter will teach us about lauric acid and about good cholesterol and bad cholesterol.

Coconut Milk, Cholesterol and Blood Pressure

Since coconuts are a great source of lauric acid they assist in lowering blood pressure and cholesterol. There are several studies that show lauric acid is a protective type of fatty acid connected with better heart health and good cholesterol levels.

In one study 60 healthy volunteers drank coconut milk porridge for 8 weeks, 5 days a week. Research showed their low density lipoprotein (LDL) levels decreased while their high density lipoprotein (HDL) levels increased.

Since cholesterol can't dissolve in the blood, it has to be transported by carriers known as lipoproteins. Lipoproteins are made of fat, or lipids, and proteins. There are two types of these lipoproteins that can carry the cholesterol: low-density/LDL and high-density/HDL.

LDL cholesterol is considered detrimental because it will contribute to plaque and get stuck in the arteries and clog them up, making them less flexible and less able to carry blood. This is known as atherosclerosis. Clogged arteries can lead to heart attack and strokes.

HDL is good cholesterol because it helps to eradicate the LDL cholesterol from the arteries. Studies show HDL carries the LDL cholesterol back to the liver where it gets broken down and then removed from the body.

Somewhere between 1/4 and 1/3 of blood cholesterol is carried by HDL. Research shows that healthy levels of HDL may also help to protect the body from stroke and heart attack, while low levels of HDL increase the risk of heart disease.

The link between virgin coconut milk and healthy levels of cholesterol now becomes clear. Add in the minerals in coconut milk that are important for circulation and blood flow and you have a food that is helpful in lowering blood pressure and keeping blood vessels free from plaque and flexible.

One of the minerals in coconut milk is magnesium. The body uses magnesium to help decrease muscle tension and stress and increasing circulation. All these qualities relate to the prevention of poor heart health such as a heart attack.

Now that we've learned about how to help lower our blood pressure and cholesterol, let's find out how to make our own coconut milk at home next. There's more than one way.

Coconut Milk You Make Yourself

There's more than one way to make your own coconut milk. Now we're going to learn what those ways are.

Making Coconut Milk from a Raw Coconut

The best way I've found to make your own coconut milk is directly from a fresh coconut. First you want to start with the freshest coconut you can find. Shake it to make sure you can hear the coconut water sloshing around inside. That's a good indicator of a fresh coconut.

To crack it you'll need a sharp sturdy cleaver or heavy durable knife. If you have neither of those you can use a hammer to break it open.

Hit the top of the coconut with the cleaver (or knife or hammer) until you hear it crack. Have a measuring cup or small bowel ready and turn the coconut over to drain out the coconut water. Be sure to save the coconut water and use it for drinking, shakes, smoothies, etc.

Pry the coconut apart at the crack. At this point you'll be left with 2 or more pieces of raw coconut shell with the white meat intact inside. You can either continue hitting the shell with a hammer until the white meat pieces separate from the shell and fall out, or you can use a small knife like a paring knife to cut the white meat out and away from the shell.

Put the white coconut meat pieces in a strainer and rinse them well making sure there are no coconut shell chips attached. Now place them into your food processor, blender, etc., and add 2 cups of water. You may need more water depending on how large the coconut you started with was and how much meat it yielded. Continue blending until you get a creamy thick milk.

Now strain the mixture by pouring it out of the blender through cheesecloth or a metal strainer. This will separate out the milk from the coconut solids that didn't blend out completely. To get all the milk out, squeeze the pulp in the strainer with a large spoon or clean hands. You just made the healthiest coconut milk around!

You can use the leftover pulp in any number of ways:

Dry it for coconut flakes.

Grind the dried coconut flakes in a coffee grinder to make coconut flour.

Use it for coconut scrubs.

Add it to smoothies.

Making Coconut Milk From Dried Coconut

I've found a couple of different ways of making your own coconut milk from dried coconut. Both are very simple and take less time than making your own from a raw coconut. (However, making coconut milk from a raw coconut is my first choice.)

The first way is the simplest, but you do end up with a little grainier coconut milk. You will need:

1 cup of unsweetened dried coconut, preferably organic

4 cups of water (use filtered water, not tap water)

Blend this on high for at least 3 minutes until you get smooth, creamy milk. You'll see a nice froth on the top like you'd see on a latte. When you're satisfied with the consistency, pour it into a pitcher or a jar with a lid and store it in your refrigerator. You can also strain the mixture through cheesecloth if you want to increase the smoothness.

It will last 4-5 days when refrigerated. If it makes too much for you, just cut the recipe down.

The second way to make your own coconut milk is almost the same, but gives you smoother resulting milk. Start by putting the dried coconut in a coffee grinder and grind until it's a powder. Then proceed as above.

If not sweet enough for you, add a little of your favorite sweetener, but not too much. Some people have found that if they sweeten it they also need to add just a dash of salt.

That's it. It's super simple and so good for you. Plus, it's much easier on the pocketbook.

You've just learned how to open a raw coconut and make coconut milk at home two different ways. And you know how long it will last so you can plan ahead and know when to make the next batch.

Did you know there's another part of the coconut that has more potassium than 4 bananas and is being used instead of a sports drink? Why? We're going to find that out now in our next chapter

What Is Coconut Water and How Will It Help Me?

Here we're going to learn how important coconut water is in helping the body recover from physical exertion and how it is a great alternative to sugary sports drinks.

It is not the same as coconut milk and coconut oil. Coconut water is the clear liquid that pours out of the coconut when you first crack it. The younger the coconut, the more coconut water it contains. So look for coconuts that have a green outer shell instead of the hard brown shell often seen in grocery stores. Always shake the coconut and listen to see how much liquid is inside if you're buying for coconut water consumption.

You may recall the grueling, epic 11-hour Wimbledon tennis match won by John Isner. Says John of coconut water: "It is super hydrating and has kept me going in long matches and prevented me from cramping even in the hottest and most humid conditions." There is a reason for this.

Strenuous exercise and long periods of physical exertion cause the body to lose mineral-rich fluids. Research is showing coconut water has the same electrolyte balance found in isotonic drinks, making it valuable in rehydrating the body or bringing the body back to electrolyte balance after long periods of intensive exercise.

There are five essential electrolytes contained in coconut water that are required by the human body. They are magnesium, phosphorous, calcium, sodium and potassium. Electrolytes regulate nerve and muscle function, blood pH, blood pressure, body hydration and repair of damaged tissue in the body.

Natural coconut water has a nutty, sweet taste that is easily digestible, contains more potassium than four bananas and is cholesterol free and fat free in addition to the high electrolyte content.

Plus, there are only 5.45 calories per ounce of unflavored and unsweetened coconut water.

It is of real benefit to anyone wanting to lose weight. Due to its low fat content, dieters can drink as much as they like without worry of excessive calorie and fat consumption. Because it tastes rich, it has the tendency to make you feel full and thus suppresses the appetite, so you're filling up on the nutritious coconut water instead of calories from other sources.

You can combine coconut water with other liquids or drink it by itself. There are no set requirements or limitations on how much coconut water to drink. Since 8 ounces of coconut will have you consuming 45 to 60 calories depending on the quality, the Mayo Clinic strongly suggests you stay active if you're going to consume large quantities.

Coconut water can also be used topically for acne and skin blemishes. Topical application will tone the skin and help to clear blemishes. This is why you see a number of companies who produce facial products using coconut extract in their formulas.

Indigestion is also often aided by coconut water. Coconut water has a high concentration of fiber and not only helps to prevent indigestion and gas, but reduce the occurrence of acid reflux as well.

You just learned how to find a coconut that has the most coconut water, how to use coconut water to help you lose weight and how to use it to help clear blemishes. The final summary is next.

Conclusion

There you have it!

This book has given you the best I could find to help you start using coconut oil, coconut milk and coconut water in your daily life. Using these three coconut resources can help you:

Lose weight and burn fat.

Protect and improve brain functions.

Boost your energy.

Relax and rebuild your body.

Save money by replacing expensive products you're using now.

Make sure to try the majority of the suggestions in the book and also try to experiment with a few ideas of your own. Coconut oil is a safe, non-toxic power food and a powerful natural source of protection for your body inside and out. Adding it to your life is easy and affordable!

Taking action is probably the most important thing you can take from this book. Knowledge is not power. Applied knowledge is powerful wisdom and I want to make sure you get your money's worth for the time and energy you've spent acquiring this information.

Finally, if you enjoyed this book please take the time to share your thoughts and post a review on Amazon. It would be greatly appreciated!

Good luck and good life!

Acknowledgements

I would like to express my appreciation and gratitude to everyone who helped me complete this book, especially my mentor Angie Mroczka, whose experience and skill proved to be invaluable in getting me through a complicated process.

Many thanks to my editor, Elaine Roughton for doing such a great job so quickly and being so easy to work with.

My heartfelt gratitude to my Launch Team; I couldn't have gotten this off the ground without them and their daily support and encouragement.

A special thank you to the Facebook group Aspiring Authors and the support of all those who so willingly shared their knowledge and time to help make this book a reality.

About The Author

Raised on a small farm in the Midwest, BJ's first memories were of corn tassels, pullet eggs and watermelon cooling in the corner cistern in the kitchen. Born an introvert, the country space served her well. After chores were finished on the family farm she spent what free time there was reading and practicing piano taught by her mother.

By the time she reached her early 20's she'd migrated to the southwest where she fell in love with the mountains. After careers in Accounting and Information Technology she headed into the realm of Alternative Healing, a natural arena for her now vegan lifestyle.

As a licensed bodyworker, BJ has spent over 30 years researching, studying and practicing various types of natural healing modalities and health-related issues. She still lives in the mountains in a small rural town enjoying the seclusion and practicing her craft.

You can connect directly with BJ here:

- http://bjrichardsauthor.com/

- https://twitter.com/BJRichardsAuthr

- https://www.facebook.com/BJ.Richards.Author

ALSO: Find out about BJ's new books when they come out. Don't miss out on all the updates, revisions and new projects.

Sign up at the link below:

http://bjrichardsauthor.com/newsletter-sign-up/

Review Request

I hope you enjoyed this book as much as I enjoyed writing it. If so, would you please leave me your honest review? It would be much appreciated.

Thank you again and have a wonderful healthy life.

Made in the USA
San Bernardino, CA
08 March 2017